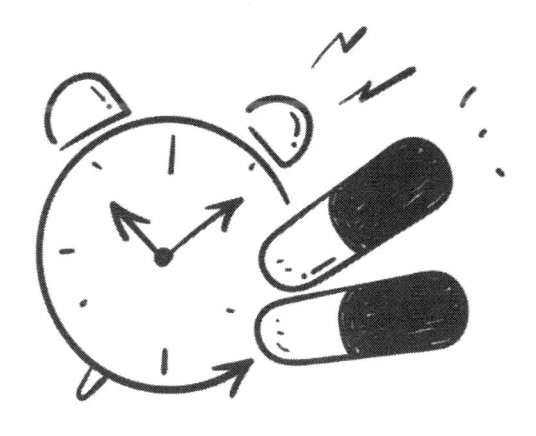

Medication

Log Book

_____

_____

_____

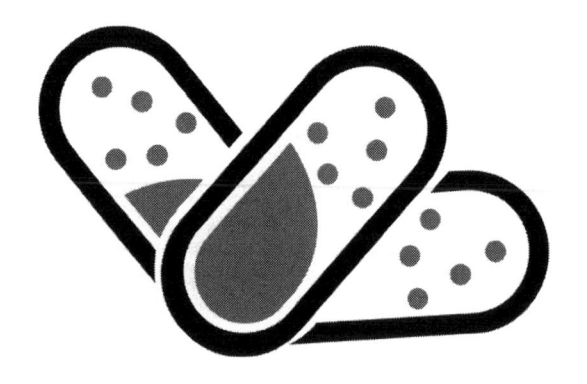

Copyright © Tarek ZA

All rights reserved

Medication Log Book

Name: Age:

Weight: Height:

Information :

Date	Time	Medication	Dose	Taken	Note

Medication Log Book

Name: Age:

Weight: Height:

Information :

Date	Time	Medication	Dose	Taken	Note

Medication Log Book

Name: Age:

Weight: Height:

Information :

Date	Time	Medication	Dose	Taken	Note

Medication Log Book

Name: Age:

Weight: Height:

Information :

Date	Time	Medication	Dose	Taken	Note

Medication Log Book

Name: Age:

Weight: Height:

Information :

Date	Time	Medication	Dose	Taken	Note

Medication Log Book

Name: Age:

Weight: Height:

Information :

Date	Time	Medication	Dose	Taken	Note

Medication Log Book

Name: Age:

Weight: Height:

Information :

Date	Time	Medication	Dose	Taken	Note

Medication Log Book

Name:　　　　　　　　　　　Age:

Weight:　　　　　　　　　　Height:

Information :

Date	Time	Medication	Dose	Taken	Note

Medication *Log Book*

Name:　　　　　　　　　　Age:

Weight:　　　　　　　　　Height:

Information :

Date	Time	Medication	Dose	Taken	Note

Medication Log Book

Name: Age:

Weight: Height:

Information :

Date	Time	Medication	Dose	Taken	Note

Medication Log Book

Name: Age:

Weight: Height:

Information :

Date	Time	Medication	Dose	Taken	Note

Medication Log Book

Name: Age:

Weight: Height:

Information :

Date	Time	Medication	Dose	Taken	Note

Medication Log Book

Name: Age:

Weight: Height:

Information :

Date	Time	Medication	Dose	Taken	Note

Medication Log Book

Name: Age:

Weight: Height:

Information :

Date	Time	Medication	Dose	Taken	Note

Medication Log Book

Name: Age:

Weight: Height:

Information :

Date	Time	Medication	Dose	Taken	Note

Medication Log Book

Name: Age:

Weight: Height:

Information :

Date	Time	Medication	Dose	Taken	Note

Medication Log Book

Name: Age:

Weight: Height:

Information :

Date	Time	Medication	Dose	Taken	Note

Medication Log Book

Name: Age:

Weight: Height:

Information :

Date	Time	Medication	Dose	Taken	Note

Medication *Log Book*

Name: Age:

Weight: Height:

Information :

Date	Time	Medication	Dose	Taken	Note

Medication Log Book

Name:　　　　　　　　　　　Age:

Weight:　　　　　　　　　　Height:

Information :

Date	Time	Medication	Dose	Taken	Note

Medication Log Book

Name: Age:

Weight: Height:

Information :

Date	Time	Medication	Dose	Taken	Note

Medication Log Book

Name: Age:

Weight: Height:

Information :

Date	Time	Medication	Dose	Taken	Note

Medication Log Book

Name: Age:

Weight: Height:

Information :

Date	Time	Medication	Dose	Taken	Note

Medication Log Book

Name: Age:

Weight: Height:

Information :

Date	Time	Medication	Dose	Taken	Note

Medication *Log Book*

Name: Age:

Weight: Height:

Information :

Date	Time	Medication	Dose	Taken	Note

Medication Log Book

Name: Age:

Weight: Height:

Information :

Date	Time	Medication	Dose	Taken	Note

Medication *Log Book*

Name: Age:

Weight: Height:

Information :

Date	Time	Medication	Dose	Taken	Note

Medication Log Book

Name: Age:

Weight: Height:

Information :

Date	Time	Medication	Dose	Taken	Note

Medication *Log Book*

Name: Age:

Weight: Height:

Information :

Date	Time	Medication	Dose	Taken	Note

Medication Log Book

Name: Age:

Weight: Height:

Information :

Date	Time	Medication	Dose	Taken	Note

Medication *Log Book*

Name: Age:

Weight: Height:

Information :

Date	Time	Medication	Dose	Taken	Note

Medication *Log Book*

Name: Age:

Weight: Height:

Information :

Date	Time	Medication	Dose	Taken	Note

Medication Log Book

Name: Age:

Weight: Height:

Information :

Date	Time	Medication	Dose	Taken	Note

Medication Log Book

Name: Age:

Weight: Height:

Information :

Date	Time	Medication	Dose	Taken	Note

Medication *Log Book*

Name: Age:

Weight: Height:

Information :

Date	Time	Medication	Dose	Taken	Note

Medication Log Book

Name: Age:

Weight: Height:

Information :

Date	Time	Medication	Dose	Taken	Note

Medication *Log Book*

Name: Age:

Weight: Height:

Information :

Date	Time	Medication	Dose	Taken	Note

Medication Log Book

Name: Age:

Weight: Height:

Information :

Date	Time	Medication	Dose	Taken	Note

Medication Log Book

Name: Age:

Weight: Height:

Information :

Date	Time	Medication	Dose	Taken	Note

Medication Log Book

Name: Age:

Weight: Height:

Information :

Date	Time	Medication	Dose	Taken	Note

Medication Log Book

Name: Age:

Weight: Height:

Information :

Date	Time	Medication	Dose	Taken	Note

Medication Log Book

Name: Age:

Weight: Height:

Information :

Date	Time	Medication	Dose	Taken	Note

Medication *Log Book*

Name: Age:

Weight: Height:

Information :

Date	Time	Medication	Dose	Taken	Note

Medication Log Book

Name: Age:

Weight: Height:

Information :

Date	Time	Medication	Dose	Taken	Note

Medication Log Book

Name: Age:

Weight: Height:

Information :

Date	Time	Medication	Dose	Taken	Note

Medication Log Book

Name: Age:

Weight: Height:

Information :

Date	Time	Medication	Dose	Taken	Note

Medication Log Book

Name: Age:

Weight: Height:

Information :

Date	Time	Medication	Dose	Taken	Note

Medication Log Book

Name: Age:

Weight: Height:

Information :

Date	Time	Medication	Dose	Taken	Note

Medication Log Book

Name: Age:

Weight: Height:

Information :

Date	Time	Medication	Dose	Taken	Note

Medication *Log Book*

Name: Age:

Weight: Height:

Information :

Date	Time	Medication	Dose	Taken	Note

Medication *Log Book*

Name: Age:

Weight: Height:

Information :

Date	Time	Medication	Dose	Taken	Note

Medication Log Book

Name: Age:

Weight: Height:

Information :

Date	Time	Medication	Dose	Taken	Note

Medication Log Book

Name: Age:

Weight: Height:

Information :

Date	Time	Medication	Dose	Taken	Note

Medication Log Book

Name: Age:

Weight: Height:

Information :

Date	Time	Medication	Dose	Taken	Note

Medication *Log Book*

Name: Age:

Weight: Height:

Information :

Date	Time	Medication	Dose	Taken	Note

Medication Log Book

Name: Age:

Weight: Height:

Information :

Date	Time	Medication	Dose	Taken	Note

Medication Log Book

Name: Age:

Weight: Height:

Information :

Date	Time	Medication	Dose	Taken	Note

Medication Log Book

Name: Age:

Weight: Height:

Information :

Date	Time	Medication	Dose	Taken	Note

Medication *Log Book*

Name: Age:

Weight: Height:

Information :

Date	Time	Medication	Dose	Taken	Note

Medication Log Book

Name: Age:

Weight: Height:

Information :

Date	Time	Medication	Dose	Taken	Note

Medication Log Book

Name: Age:

Weight: Height:

Information :

Date	Time	Medication	Dose	Taken	Note

Medication *Log Book*

Name: Age:

Weight: Height:

Information :

Date	Time	Medication	Dose	Taken	Note

Medication Log Book

Name: Age:

Weight: Height:

Information :

Date	Time	Medication	Dose	Taken	Note

Medication Log Book

Name: Age:

Weight: Height:

Information :

Date	Time	Medication	Dose	Taken	Note

Medication *Log Book*

Name: Age:

Weight: Height:

Information :

Date	Time	Medication	Dose	Taken	Note

Medication Log Book

Name: Age:

Weight: Height:

Information :

Date	Time	Medication	Dose	Taken	Note

Medication Log Book

Name: Age:

Weight: Height:

Information :

Date	Time	Medication	Dose	Taken	Note

Medication Log Book

Name: Age:

Weight: Height:

Information :

Date	Time	Medication	Dose	Taken	Note

Medication Log Book

Name: Age:

Weight: Height:

Information :

Date	Time	Medication	Dose	Taken	Note

Medication *Log Book*

Name: Age:

Weight: Height:

Information :

Date	Time	Medication	Dose	Taken	Note

Medication *Log Book*

Name: Age:

Weight: Height:

Information :

Date	Time	Medication	Dose	Taken	Note

＃ Medication Log Book

Name: Age:

Weight: Height:

Information :

Date	Time	Medication	Dose	Taken	Note

Medication Log Book

Name: Age:

Weight: Height:

Information :

Date	Time	Medication	Dose	Taken	Note

Medication *Log Book*

Name: Age:

Weight: Height:

Information :

Date	Time	Medication	Dose	Taken	Note

Medication *Log Book*

Name: Age:

Weight: Height:

Information :

Date	Time	Medication	Dose	Taken	Note

Medication Log Book

Name: Age:

Weight: Height:

Information :

Date	Time	Medication	Dose	Taken	Note

Medication *Log Book*

Name: Age:

Weight: Height:

Information :

Date	Time	Medication	Dose	Taken	Note

Medication Log Book

Name:　　　　　　　　　　　Age:

Weight:　　　　　　　　　　Height:

Information :

Date	Time	Medication	Dose	Taken	Note

Medication *Log Book*

Name: Age:

Weight: Height:

Information :

Date	Time	Medication	Dose	Taken	Note

Medication Log Book

Name: Age:

Weight: Height:

Information :

Date	Time	Medication	Dose	Taken	Note

Medication Log Book

Name: Age:

Weight: Height:

Information :

Date	Time	Medication	Dose	Taken	Note

Medication *Log Book*

Name:　　　　　　　　　　　Age:

Weight:　　　　　　　　　　Height:

Information :

Date	Time	Medication	Dose	Taken	Note

Medication Log Book

Name: Age:

Weight: Height:

Information :

Date	Time	Medication	Dose	Taken	Note

Medication Log Book

Name: Age:

Weight: Height:

Information :

Date	Time	Medication	Dose	Taken	Note

Medication *Log Book*

Name: Age:

Weight: Height:

Information :

Date	Time	Medication	Dose	Taken	Note

Medication Log Book

Name: Age:

Weight: Height:

Information :

Date	Time	Medication	Dose	Taken	Note

Medication *Log Book*

Name: Age:

Weight: Height:

Information :

Date	Time	Medication	Dose	Taken	Note

Medication *Log Book*

Name: Age:

Weight: Height:

Information :

Date	Time	Medication	Dose	Taken	Note

Medication Log Book

Name:	Age:

Weight:	Height:

Information :

Date	Time	Medication	Dose	Taken	Note

Medication Log Book

Name: Age:

Weight: Height:

Information :

Date	Time	Medication	Dose	Taken	Note

Medication *Log Book*

Name: Age:

Weight: Height:

Information :

Date	Time	Medication	Dose	Taken	Note

Medication Log Book

Name:	Age:

Weight:	Height:

Information :

Date	Time	Medication	Dose	Taken	Note

Medication *Log Book*

Name: Age:

Weight: Height:

Information :

Date	Time	Medication	Dose	Taken	Note

Medication *Log Book*

Name: Age:

Weight: Height:

Information :

Date	Time	Medication	Dose	Taken	Note

Medication Log Book

Name: Age:

Weight: Height:

Information :

Date	Time	Medication	Dose	Taken	Note

Medication *Log Book*

Name: Age:

Weight: Height:

Information :

Date	Time	Medication	Dose	Taken	Note

Medication *Log Book*

Name: Age:

Weight: Height:

Information :

Date	Time	Medication	Dose	Taken	Note

Medication *Log Book*

Name: Age:

Weight: Height:

Information :

Date	Time	Medication	Dose	Taken	Note

Medication Log Book

Name: Age:

Weight: Height:

Information :

Date	Time	Medication	Dose	Taken	Note

Medication Log Book

Name: Age:

Weight: Height:

Information :

Date	Time	Medication	Dose	Taken	Note

Medication *Log Book*

Name: Age:

Weight: Height:

Information :

Date	Time	Medication	Dose	Taken	Note

Medication *Log Book*

Name: Age:

Weight: Height:

Information :

Date	Time	Medication	Dose	Taken	Note

Medication Log Book

Name: Age:

Weight: Height:

Information :

Date	Time	Medication	Dose	Taken	Note

Medication Log Book

Name: Age:

Weight: Height:

Information :

Date	Time	Medication	Dose	Taken	Note

Medication *Log Book*

Name:　　　　　　　　　　　Age:

Weight:　　　　　　　　　　Height:

Information :

Date	Time	Medication	Dose	Taken	Note

Medication *Log Book*

Name:　　　　　　　　　　　Age:

Weight:　　　　　　　　　　Height:

Information :

Date	Time	Medication	Dose	Taken	Note

Medication Log Book

Name: Age:

Weight: Height:

Information :

Date	Time	Medication	Dose	Taken	Note

Medication *Log Book*

Name: Age:

Weight: Height:

Information :

Date	Time	Medication	Dose	Taken	Note

Medication *Log Book*

Name: Age:

Weight: Height:

Information :

Date	Time	Medication	Dose	Taken	Note

Medication Log Book

Name: Age:

Weight: Height:

Information :

Date	Time	Medication	Dose	Taken	Note

Medication Log Book

Name: Age:

Weight: Height:

Information :

Date	Time	Medication	Dose	Taken	Note

Medication Log Book

Name: Age:

Weight: Height:

Information :

Date	Time	Medication	Dose	Taken	Note

Medication Log Book

Name: Age:

Weight: Height:

Information :

Date	Time	Medication	Dose	Taken	Note

Medication *Log Book*

Name: Age:

Weight: Height:

Information :

Date	Time	Medication	Dose	Taken	Note

Medication *Log Book*

Name: Age:

Weight: Height:

Information :

Date	Time	Medication	Dose	Taken	Note

Medication *Log Book*

Name: Age:

Weight: Height:

Information :

Date	Time	Medication	Dose	Taken	Note

Medication Log Book

Name: Age:

Weight: Height:

Information :

Date	Time	Medication	Dose	Taken	Note

Medication Log Book

Name: Age:

Weight: Height:

Information :

Date	Time	Medication	Dose	Taken	Note

Printed in Great Britain
by Amazon

75c6fb13-4c32-4373-a33b-37b996bfbb09R01